50 Green Smoothie Diet Recipes!

Green Smoothie Diet

The Ultimate 5-Day Detox Dieting Guide To Improve Health, Boost Energy, Lose Weight, Kick Cravings, And Rejuvenate With Essential Smoothies!

Chris Smith

STOP!!! Before you read any further....Would you like to know the Secrets of Body Transformation?

If your answer is yes, then you are not alone. Thousands of people are looking for the secret to rapidly burn body fat, keep the weight off, become healthier, and truly transform their body and life for good.

If you have been searching for these answers without much luck, you are in the right place!

Not only will you gain incredible insight in this book, but because I want to make sure to give you as much value as possible, right now for a limited time you can get full **100% FREE access to a VIP bonus EBook** entitled **THE 7 KEYS TO BODY TRANSFORMATION!**

Just Go Here For Free Instant Access:

www.liveFitVIP.com

Legal Notice

Disclaimer Notice

Table Of Contents

Introduction

I want to thank you and congratulate you for purchasing the book, *"50 Green Smoothie Diet Recipes! - The Ultimate 5 Day Detox Dieting Guide To Improve Health, Boost Energy, Lose Weight, Kick Cravings, And Rejuvenate With Essential Smoothies!"*.

This "Green Smoothie Diet" book contains proven steps and strategies on how to heal your body, fight diseases, eliminate existing medical conditions, enhance your immunity, lose weight, regain your energy, improve your mood, jump start your metabolism, get rid of your cravings, fight the signs of aging, and achieve overall health and wellness by going on the Green Smoothie Diet.

You will learn how to do all these in just five days. Each day, you will focus on a specific benefit of the Green Smoothie Diet and learn how to make green smoothie recipes specifically formulated with that day's health focus in mind. At the end of five days, you will have detoxified your body, shed some pounds, gave your energy level a boost, and felt the immediate beneficial effects of super healing foods to your health and wellbeing.

This comprehensive guide contains tips and tricks on the proper preparation, consumption and storage of green smoothies. It also shows you how to make your smoothies extra scrumptious, how to get the optimum amount of nutrients from your smoothies, and how to make them in less time. Best of all, this book offers you 50 delicious and nutritious green smoothies to get you started on your diet! Excited? Flip the page and start now!

Thanks again for purchasing this book, I hope you enjoy it!

Chapter 1: What Is The Green Smoothie Diet?

Green smoothies have gone well past just being a diet trend. Today, many people know about their health benefits and are regular green smoothie drinkers. They aren't hard to find anymore either, as many cafes, restaurants, and juice bars now offer various green smoothie concoctions. Nutritionists and dieticians have acknowledged the beneficial effects of green smoothies, and there are thousands of articles on the Internet touting the healing powers of these amazing drinks.

Green Smoothies vs. "Green Smoothies"

However, before we discuss the Green Smoothie Diet, let's get one thing straight: overpriced, artificially sweetened drinks disguised as "green smoothies" are not the same as *real*, homemade, 100% natural green smoothies. The real deal does not contain artificial sweeteners, refined sugar, food coloring, ice cream and juice concentrates. Real, honest-to-goodness, health-boosting green smoothies are made with only the freshest, preferably organic vegetables and fruits blended together with well-chosen all-natural superfoods such as Spirulina and chia seeds. Unlike store-bought smoothies, there is no place in a real green smoothie for high fructose corn syrup or food dyes.

The Green Smoothie Diet

The challenge behind the Green Smoothie Diet is to drink at least one green smoothie a day. The reason behind it is that regular consumption of green smoothies helps you lose weight, makes you feel more energetic, improves your immunity, gives you a youthful glow, treats or reduces the symptoms of existing health issues, cleanses your body and just gives you an overall feeling of good health from the inside out.

Considerations

Green smoothies are great meal replacements, but replacing *all* your meals with smoothies is not recommended. These drinks, though nutrient-dense, do not have enough calories in them to replace your every meal. Anything that has fewer than 300 calories is not a fit meal. For best results, replace your breakfast and one other light meal (e.g. your afternoon snack) with a green smoothie. Any more than that and you are starving yourself.

Chapter 2: Health Benefits Of The Green Smoothie Diet

For something that is so easy to make, the humble green smoothie offers so many different health benefits. Depending on what ingredients you put into it, a green smoothie can

(1) aid in weight loss,
(2) boost energy,
(3) detoxify the body,
(4) improve one's mood,
(5) enhance immunity,
(6) heal or reduce the effects of existing health conditions, and
(7) all of the above.

Regardless of the intended purpose of a green smoothie recipe, it is sure to nourish the body. All green smoothies offer mega doses of vitamins, minerals, micronutrients and healthy fats that are essential to the proper functioning of the body and to overall health and wellness.

What can green smoothies do for you?

• Green smoothies are detoxifying.

Because of the fruit and vegetable content of green smoothies, these wholesome drinks provide loads of vitamins, minerals and fiber that cleanse the body and reverse the signs of aging. Taking green smoothies regularly makes your skin and hair glow, allows your internal organs to function as though you were years younger, and leaves you feeling rejuvenated.

• Green smoothies are energy-boosting.

If you find that you can't function without your daily dose/s of caffeine, but know that drinking too much coffee is bad for you, switch to green smoothies. Green smoothies have an uplifting effect on one's mood and enable one to perform strongly throughout the workday without the excess sugars and fats in most caffeinated drinks.

• Green smoothies are slimming.

Green smoothies help aid weight loss in a number of ways. First, the fiber in fresh fruits and vegetables, that are incorporated in the smoothie and not tossed out (as in green juices), helps flush out fats from the body. Second, fruits and vegetables contain enzymes that literally melt away fats. Third, green smoothies are excellent meal replacements. They can leave you just as satisfied as if you had eaten a full meal, but without all the unhealthy carbohydrates and fats that you would consume in a typical meal. Believe it or not, a green smoothie can even satiate a craving for sweets.

- Green smoothies are disease fighting.

Fresh fruits and vegetables, consumed in their raw, unprocessed forms, are rich in vitamins, minerals, phytonutrients, amino acids, antioxidants, and beneficial enzymes that protect you against illness and help treat current health problems.

Chapter 3: Day 1 – How To Heal Your Body Using Healing Foods

Having your daily green smoothie is like supercharging yourself with the full healing powers of Mother Nature.

Fresh fruits, vegetables, and herbs – the basic ingredients of a green smoothie – are chockfull of live enzymes that rid the body of toxins and other harmful chemicals. Detoxification allows the body to improve its functions, reenergize, and get much-needed rest from the onslaught of excess fats, sugars, artificial ingredients, and chemicals such as pesticides and fertilizers in our food, as well as the many pollutants in our environment. For those who live particularly unhealthy lifestyles, detoxifying every once in a while is essential. Regular consumption of green smoothies is a great way to detoxify. These green smoothie ingredients have highly potent detoxifying properties:

- Leafy green vegetables such as kale, lettuce, spinach, collard greens, celery and bokchoy are loaded with fiber that literally scrubs out your intestines. They are also rich in protein and flavonoids. Spinach is a great source of Vitamin K, Vitamin A, iron and magnesium. Parsley is a known diuretic. The glucosinates in kale facilitate detoxification at the genetic level.
- Cilantro has been found effective in ridding the body of metals such as mercury.
- Basil is a diuretic and has antimicrobial, anti-ulcer and anticancer properties.
- Berries are packed with antioxidants that prevent free radical damage.
- Seeds such as chia and flax, and nuts such as almond and sunflower, are loaded with vitamins and good fats.
- Apples are rich in pectin, a soluble fiber that helps eliminate food additives and heavy metals from the body.
- Avocados have glutathione, which aid the liver in removing harmful chemicals from the body.
- Pineapples are rich in bromelain, an enzyme that helps the digestive and excretory systems.

Recipes 1-10 in Chapter 8: 50 Amazing Green Smoothie Diet Recipes were formulated to help you detoxify your body and thus boost its natural ability to heal itself.

Chapter 4: Day 2 – How To Fight Diseases And Diabetes Using Green Smoothies

It's true: a green smoothie a day can keep the doctor away. Dozens of scientific studies proved that regular consumption of adequate servings of fresh, raw vegetables and fruits helps fend off the onset of the so-called lifestyle diseases: cancer, cardiovascular illness, diabetes, obesity, osteoporosis, kidney trouble, depression, and more. Drinking a green smoothie every day is the easiest and fastest way to make sure that you are getting the number of suggested daily servings of fruits and vegetables and of the required daily values of essential vitamins and minerals.

How do green smoothies help you fight diseases?

- A diet rich in whole vegetables and fruits helps prevent and even reverse cardiovascular diseases, cancer, diabetes, obesity, Alzheimer's, kidney disease, osteoporosis and many other illnesses.
- Plant-based foods that are filling enough to replace a typical meat-based meal reduce the amount of animal fats and animal protein in the body, thus facilitating weight loss and preventing obesity and related diseases.
- Drinks with non-dairy bases are better for you because they are less fattening, but may even be more nutritious. This is especially true for green smoothies that contain calcium-rich fruits and vegetables. Certain studies have even linked regular dairy consumption to higher rates of osteoporosis and fractures.
- Plant-rich or plant-based foods such as green smoothies have just as much or even more protein than animal foods, but are more nutrient-dense and have fewer or zero cholesterol. Consuming a diet rich in plant-based foods promotes cardiovascular health.

Recipes 11-20 in Chapter 8: 50 Amazing Green Smoothie Diet Recipes were formulated to help strengthen your body's immune system and thus prevent illness.

Chapter 5: Day 3 – How To Improve Mood And Boost Energy Using Green Smoothies

Millions of people have a dangerous coffee habit that they believe they can't escape. If you are one of these people, then you probably feel like you can't make it through the morning without your regular latte (or other caffeinated drink). Once the mid-day slump hits you, you reach for another cup. Most people with a coffee habit consume at least five cups of coffee throughout the day, with some drinking as many as nine or 10 cups.

By now, we know that some amount of coffee consumed daily may not be all that bad and may even have beneficial effects for the brain and the heart. However, an excess of caffeine is definitely not good and may lead to heart palpitations, nutrient imbalances, bone loss and leaky gut syndrome. The sugar and dairy we add to coffee contributes to obesity, diabetes, cardiovascular disease, and many other health problems.

You can replace your morning cup of coffee and still get a boost of energy and a natural high that will take you through an arduous workday. Yes, and when you drink a green smoothie instead of a cappuccino, you decrease the amount of calories you consume, get a huge dose of vitamins and minerals, *and* get an energy boost that will last *the whole day*.

Green smoothies help enhance your mood too, because the vitamins and minerals in the fresh fruits and vegetables in your glass of green goodness are rich in fiber. Fiber flushes out environmental estrogen that causes hormonal imbalance, making you act out in ways that are "estrogen dominant". Green smoothies also contain iron, magnesium, and Vitamin B, all of which help balance your hormones and drive away those depressing doldrums.

Recipes 21-30 in Chapter 8: 50 Amazing Green Smoothie Diet Recipes were formulated to help reduce your mood swings, give you more energy and make you more optimistic, focused and vibrant.

Chapter 6: Day 4 – Lose Weight And Get In Shape With Green Smoothies

If you have been trying all kinds of diets and cleanses without seeing any results, a green smoothie just might do the trick. Perhaps, it is now time for you to go on the Green Smoothie Diet.

Why? Because green smoothies help you shed the pounds in several ways.

First, it's great as a meal replacement. Unlike the juices that you take on a juice diet, smoothies have more bulk and are thus more filling, leaving your tummy sated for longer, so you don't return to the fridge every 15 minutes. And because you can make your green smoothie without any animal products whatsoever, it is perfect for vegetarians and for vegans. Taking a green smoothie or green "thickie" leaves you with the same full-tummy feeling as when you indulge in a favorite snack or even a full meal. However, the green smoothie has significantly fewer calories and no added fats and sugars.

Second, green smoothies are made with fresh fruits and vegetables. The dietary fibers in these promote weight loss and even help prevent weight gain. Recently, a study in the *Journal of Nutrition* found that increasing fiber intake by 8 grams for every 1000 calories consumed resulted in a weight loss of about 4 ½ pounds.

Third, the fruits and vegetables that make up a green smoothie are high in critically important vitamins, minerals, and enzymes that promote the burning of accumulated fats in the body.

Fourth, fruits and vegetables are naturally low in calories, but high in nutrients. If you are used to a diet of carbohydrates, sugars, fats and salt, going on the Green Smoothie Diet will be a pleasant break for your system and an easy, effortless way to naturally reduce the number of calories you consume every day.

Recipes 31-40 in Chapter 8: 50 Amazing Green Smoothie Diet Recipes were formulated to help you lose pounds and tone your body without taking pills or exercising.

Chapter 7: Day 5 – Jump Start Your Metabolism With Green Smoothies

If you are overweight, constantly tired, chronically stressed, and sleep-deprived, you need to make green smoothies a part of your daily routine.

The green smoothie is an ideal weight loss tool, especially for those who have struggled long and hard trying to lose weight. It gives your metabolism a boost, helping you lose weight while preventing weight gain, BUT it doesn't leave you feeling deprived.

How do green smoothies give your metabolism a boost? Green smoothies are made with ingredients that are incredible metabolism boosters.

- Water is one of the best natural appetite suppressants. Drinking a bottle of water raises your metabolism by about 30%.
- Leafy green vegetables help stabilize your blood sugar levels, which in turn helps prevent the conversion of excess sugars into body fat.
- Celery is a known thermogenic food, is low in calories, and has high levels of calcium.
- Cruciferous vegetables such as broccoli, cauliflower, Brussels sprouts and cabbage contain phytonutrients, are low in calories and are high in fiber. Studies also show that cruciferous vegetables are able to restore the balance in estrogen metabolism and thus facilitate body fat loss, especially in the abdominal area.
- Blueberries are rich in flavonoids that support metabolism by allowing the leptins in our bodies to function properly.
- Citrus fruits, with their rich Vitamin C content, are excellent fat burners and help speed up metabolism.
- Melons are loaded with potassium, which is essential in the liver's work of making glycogen. The release of glycogen into the bloodstream prevents the slowing down of your metabolism.
- Avocados are rich in omega-3 fatty acids that are crucial to metabolism.

Recipes 41-50 in Chapter 8: 50 Amazing Green Smoothie Diet Recipes were formulated to help get your metabolism going, thus giving you more energy and preventing the conversion of excess oils and sugars in your diet into fats.

Chapter 8: 50 Amazing Green Smoothie Diet Recipes

Healing Smoothies

1. Simple Green Smoothie

This is the basic recipe for green smoothies. Build on it by adding different combinations of greens and non-starchy fruits.

- 1 mango, cubed
- 1 banana, sliced and frozen
- 3-4 handfuls of lettuce or spinach or other green, leafy vegetable
- a little bit of water to thin down the smoothie (optional)

Start the smoothie by placing the frozen banana slices in the blender with a bit of water. Puree. Add the mangoes and blend. Add the greens and blend to the desired consistency. If the smoothie is too thick, add a tablespoon or so of water and pulse a few times. Serve immediately.

2. Rawmazing Green Smoothie

A mix of super healthy fruits and vegetables, this green smoothie packs a powerful health-boosting punch.

- 1 banana, sliced and frozen
- 1 cup mixed berries, fresh or frozen
- a handful of spinach
- a handful of celery
- a handful of parsley
- 1 orange mint leaf
- water (optional)

Blend the banana, berries and water (add a tablespoon at a time) together. Add the spinach, celery, parsley and mint. Blend to the desired consistency. Serve with a mint garnish.

3. Health Warrior Green Smoothie

Get on the path to becoming a health warrior by making this delicious green smoothie a part of your daily diet.

- 2 cups mango, cubed
- 1 ½ cups kale, chopped
- ½ cup parsley
- 1 celery stalk, sliced
- 1 cup fresh-squeezed orange or apple juice

Blend the mango and juice until the fruit is pureed. Add the kale, parsley and celery. Blend to the desired consistency. Serve immediately.

4. Complete Cleansing Tropical Smoothie

Who says detox drinks have to be tasteless or disgusting? Try this certified yummy smoothie bursting with tropical fruit flavors and you'll be hooked!

- 1 frozen banana, sliced and frozen
- 1 mango, cubed
- 1 cup fresh coconut water (if unavailable, substitute with water)
- 1 inch fresh ginger, peeled and grated
- 3 cups assorted leafy greens
- 1/4teaspoon Spirulina
- ½ teaspoon moringa powder
- 1/8 teaspoon cayenne pepper
- ½ teaspoon organic coco sugar or 1 teaspoon raw honey
- chia seeds (optional)
- ice cubes (optional)

Blend the banana, mango, ginger, coconut water and ice together until the solids have mostly pureed. Add the greens, spirulina, cayenne pepper, moringa powder, and sweetener. Blend to the desired consistency. Mix in the chia seeds and serve immediately.

5. Super Veggie Green Smoothie

What better way is there to make sure that you're getting your daily dose of fresh vegetables than by drinking them all in one go?

- 5-6 broccoli florets, chopped
- 1 frozen banana, sliced and frozen
- 1 apple, cubed
- 1 cup spinach
- 1 cup Romaine lettuce
- 1 cup fresh-squeezed orange or apple juice

- 1 teaspoon honey (optional)

Blend the banana with the apple, broccoli and juice. Add the spinach, lettuce and sweetener. Blend to the desired consistency. Serve immediately.

6. Total Immunity Green Smoothie

You'll enjoy sipping this deceptively sweet (but unsweetened!) smoothie so much, you can almost forget that it's giving your immune system a much-needed boost!

- 1 cup papaya, cubed
- 1 banana, sliced and frozen
- 1 cup strawberries, sliced
- 2-3 handfuls of spinach or kale
- a handful of parsley
- 1 celery stalk, sliced
- ice cubes

Process the banana, strawberries, papaya and ice until well-blended. Add the greens, celery and parsley. Blend to the desired consistency. Garnish with a strawberry slice and serve immediately.

7. Goddess of Greens Super Smoothie

Get youthful, glowing skin and fight the signs of aging with this chlorophyll-rich green smoothie.

- ½ head Romaine lettuce
- 2 handfuls parsley
- 2 celery stalks, sliced
- 2 handfuls of spinach
- a handful of coriander (if coriander is not to your liking, replace with equal amount of other green herb or leafy green)
- 1 banana, sliced and frozen
- 1 pear, cubed
- 1 apple, cubed
- 2-3 tablespoons lemon juice

Blend the banana, pear and apple together. Add the Romaine lettuce and pulse a few times. Add the parsley, celery, spinach, coriander and lemon juice. Blend to the desired consistency. Garnish with a celery stalk and serve immediately.

8. "Banish Inflammation" Green Smoothie

Inflammation in the body is the cause of many so-called lifestyle diseases, i.e. cancer, diabetes and cardiovascular problems. Eliminate inflammation by loading up on this smoothie.

- 2 cups assorted leafy greens
- a handful of parsley
- 1 banana, sliced and frozen
- 1 cucumber, peeled and sliced
- 1 ½ cups fresh pineapple, cubed
- ½-inch fresh ginger, peeled and grated
- 1 cup fresh coconut water or plain water
- ice cubes (optional)

Process the pineapple, banana, ginger, coconut water and ice together until well-blended. Add the cucumber and pulse a few times. Add the greens and the parsley. Blend to the desired consistency. Garnish with a pineapple wedge and serve immediately.

9. Hulk Juice

Make this truly *green* smoothie and tell anyone who asks that it's a secret potion that will turn you into a gigantic green Avenger.

- ½ cup avocado, cubed
- ½ mango, cubed
- 3-4 handfuls assorted leafy greens
- ¼ cup celery, sliced
- 1 tablespoon fresh-squeezed lime
- ½ cup water
- ice cubes (optional)

Blend the avocado, mango, water and ice together. Add the greens, celery and lime. Blend to the desired consistency. Serve with a lime wedge.

10. The King of All Smoothies

This smoothie has potent healing and rejuvenating powers. It is packed with fruits, vegetables and superfood supplements, giving it mega doses of essential vitamins and minerals, amino acids and electrolytes.

- 2 bananas, sliced and frozen

- 1 mango, cubed
- 1 kiwi, sliced
- ¼ cup dragonfruit, cubed
- 1 cup kale
- 1 cup Romaine lettuce
- 1 cup spinach
- ¼ teaspoon spirulina
- ¼ teaspoon maca powder
- 2 cups fresh coconut water (if unavailable, substitute with water)
- 1 teaspoon honey (only if the smoothie is lacking in sweetness)
- a sprinkle of chia seeds
- a sprinkle of golden flax seeds
- ice cubes (optional)

Blend the bananas, mango, kiwi, dragonfruit, coconut water and ice together. Add the kale, Romaine lettuce, spinach, honey, maca powder, spirulina, flax seeds and chia seeds. Blend to the desired consistency. Serve with a sprinkling of more chia seeds on top.

Disease-Fighting Smoothies

11. The Green Wizard

Green apples are excellent sources of Vitamin A, Vitamin C and calcium while cucumbers are rich in Vitamin K, potassium and manganese.

- 1 green apple, cubed
- 1 cucumber, peeled and sliced
- 1 mango, cubed
- 2 handfuls lettuce
- juice of 1 lemon
- 1 teaspoon moringa powder
- 1 teaspoon spirulina
- 1 cup water

Blend the apple, cucumber, mango and water together. Add the lettuce, lemon juice, moringa powder and spirulina. Blend to the desired consistency. Garnish with a cucumber slice and serve immediately.

12. Valentine's Day Green Smoothie

Red fruits and vegetables are rich in antioxidants such as anthocyanins and lycopene. These help ward off a plethora of diseases, from prostate cancer to heart disease.

- 3 handfuls red endive leaves
- 1 cup dark red cherries, fresh or frozen
- 1 teaspoon honey or ½ teaspoon organic coco sugar
- 1 teaspoon chia seeds
- 1 tablespoon raw cacao powder
- 1 cup water

Blend the cherries and the water. Add the endive leaves, honey, chia seeds and cacao powder. Blend to the desired consistency. Top with a sprinkling of cacao powder and serve immediately.

13. Rawnana Delight Smoothie

Bananas are rich in potassium, magnesium and Vitamin A, while flax seeds are packed with omega-3 essential fatty acids and fiber. Together, these two superfood ingredients make a delightful drink reminiscent of heavenly banana bread.

- 3 bananas, sliced and frozen
- 3 tablespoons golden flax seeds
- 5 Medjool dates, pitted
- 2 cups water
- ice cubes

Process the bananas, dates, flax seeds, water and ice until well-blended and smooth. Sprinkle with more flax seeds and serve immediately.

14. Very Berrylicious Green Smoothie

Berries pack a vibrant nutritional punch in this berry-centered smoothie.

- 2 cups mixed berries, fresh or frozen
- 2 handfuls kale
- ½-inch fresh ginger, peeled and grated
- ¼ teaspoon camucamu berry
- 1 teaspoon honey or ½ teaspoon organic coco sugar
- 1 tablespoon goji berries
- juice of half a lemon
- 1 cup water

Blend the berries, kale, ginger, and water. Add the camucamu berry, goji berries, sweetener and lemon juice. Blend to the desired consistency. Top with more fresh berries or goji berries and serve immediately.

15. The Purple Monster
Purple is another vivid hue that signals that a fruit or vegetable is loaded with antioxidants.

- 1 cup blueberries, fresh or frozen
- 1 banana, sliced and frozen
- 1 cup spinach
- 1 cup fresh-squeezed orange juice
- 1 teaspoon honey or ½ teaspoon organic coconut sugar

Blend the blueberries, banana, and orange juice together. Add the spinach and the sweetener. Blend to the desired consistency. Top with more blueberries and serve immediately.

16. Quick Vitamin Boost Smoothie
This basic but nutrient-packed smoothie requires only four ingredients.

- 1 banana, sliced and frozen
- 10 strawberries, fresh or frozen
- a handful of kale
- water

Process everything together until well-blended and smooth. Garnish with a strawberry slice and serve immediately.

17. Sweet Summer Smoothie
This is as decadent as your favorite fat-loaded milkshake, but without the unnecessary calories.

- 1 banana, sliced and frozen
- ½ cup blueberries, fresh or frozen
- ½ avocado, cubed
- ½ head Romaine lettuce
- Water

Process the banana, blueberries, avocado and water together until well-blended. Add the Romaine lettuce and blend to the desired consistency. Garnish with a mint leaf and serve immediately.

18. "Good For Your Gut" Green Smoothie
Keep your tummy happy and sip on this delightful smoothie.

- 1 cup papaya, cubed
- 1 cup spinach
- handful of parsley
- 1 teaspoon honey
- water

Blend the papaya and water together until pureed. Add the spinach, parsley and honey. Blend to the desired consistency. Serve immediately.

19. Divine Sweets Green Smoothie
Trick your taste buds with this sweet and sinful all-day drink.

- 1 cup blueberries, fresh or frozen
- 1 cup spinach
- 1 cup peaches, pitted
- 1 teaspoon honey or ½ teaspoon organic coco sugar
- water

Process the blueberries, peaches and water together. Add the spinach and sweetener and pulse some more. Serve immediately.

20. Fruit Fiesta Smoothie

This smoothie features four different fruits for mega doses of essential vitamins and minerals.

- 1 banana, sliced and frozen
- 1 kiwi, sliced
- ½ cup strawberries, halved
- ½ cup blueberries, fresh or frozen
- ½ head Romaine lettuce
- 2 handfuls spinach
- 1 celery stalk
- water

Blend the banana, strawberries, kiwi, blueberries and water together. Add the lettuce, spinach and celery. Blend to the desired consistency. Garnish with fresh fruit and serve immediately.

Mood- and Energy-Boosting Smoothies

21. Good Morning Smoothie
Start the day right with this energizing non-caffeinated drink.

- 3 handfuls Romaine lettuce
- 1 apple, cubed
- ½ cucumber, peeled and sliced
- ½ avocado, cubed (if unavailable, substitute with raw almond butter or non-dairy milk)
- 1 Medjool date, pitted
- a handful of parsley or cilantro
- water

Blend the apple, avocado, cucumber and water together. Add the lettuce, date and parsley/cilantro. Blend to the desired consistency. Serve immediately.

22. "It's Gonna Be A Busy Day" Green Smoothie
Fuel up before the morning rush with this energizing smoothie that you can make in a jiffy.

- 1 banana, sliced and frozen
- 1 cup kale
- 1 cup coconut water
- 1 tablespoon virgin coconut oil
- 2 tablespoons cacao nibs
- 1 teaspoon honey
- 1 scoop hemp protein powder
- 1 tablespoon chia seeds

Blend the banana with the coconut water. Add the kale, VCO, cacao nibs, honey, hemp protein powder and chia seeds. Blend to the desired consistency. Serve immediately or pour in a tumbler and drink on the go.

23. Power-Up Strawberry Smoothie
Get an energy boost and a hit of flavorful goodness to power you up for the day.

- 1 banana, sliced and frozen
- ½ cup strawberries, halved
- 3 Medjool dates, pitted
- 1 cup spinach
- 1 cup water
- 1 tablespoon golden flax seeds

- ice cubes

Process the banana, strawberries, dates, water and ice. Add the spinach and flax seeds. Blend to the desired consistency. Serve immediately.

24. Rise-and-Shine Green Smoothie

Ginger adds a nice zing to this smoothie – the perfect flavor to perk up your spirits in the morning.

- 1 banana, sliced and frozen
- 1 cup assorted leafy greens
- ½ teaspoon fresh ginger, peeled and grated
- 1 teaspoon honey
- water

Blend the banana with the water. Add the greens, ginger, and honey. Blend to the desired consistency. Serve while cold.

25. Choco Banana Waker-Upper

Who says you can't have dessert for breakfast? This smoothie gives you energy and satisfies your cravings at the same time.

- 1 banana, sliced and frozen
- 1 cup spinach
- 2 tablespoons raw cocoa powder
- 1 cup water
- 1 teaspoon virgin coconut oil
- ice cubes
- cacao nibs

Process the banana, water and ice. Add the spinach, cocoa powder and VCO. Blend to the desired consistency. Serve immediately.

26. Morning Madness Green Smoothie

What better way to start the daily grind than to indulge in a scrumptious breakfast that's chockfull of healthy goodness? Sip this smoothie and be the master of the morning rush.

- 1 banana, sliced and frozen
- ½ cup grapes, halved
- 1 apple, cubed
- 2 handfuls Romaine lettuce
- 2 celery stalks

- ¼ teaspoon spirulina
- 1 teaspoon honey (optional)
- water

Process the banana, apple, grapes, and water. Add the lettuce, celery, and spirulina. Add honey to taste. Blend to the desired consistency. Serve immediately.

27. Banana-Pineapple Surprise

Activate your "feel good" hormones with a decadent morning drink.

- 1 banana, sliced and frozen
- 1 cup fresh pineapple, cubed
- a handful of kale
- a handful of parsley
- 1 cup fresh pineapple juice
- ice cubes
- 1 teaspoon honey (optional)

Blend the banana, pineapple, juice and ice together. Add the kale, parsley and honey. Blend to the desired consistency. Serve while cold.

28. Quick Tropical Treat

Get a mood boost with an easy-to-prepare green smoothie with the taste of the islands and the goodness of tropical fruits.

- ½ papaya, cubed
- 1 banana, sliced and frozen
- 1 cup spinach
- 1 teaspoon honey
- 1 orange mint leaf
- water
- ice cubes

Blend the banana and the papaya with the water and the ice. Add the spinach, honey and mint. Pulse some more. Serve while cold.

29. Green Latte

Your daily green smoothie *can* replace your morning cuppa. A bit of healthy fat gives you an energy boost that will sustain you for the rest of the morning.

- 1 avocado, cubed

- a handful of kale
- a handful of parsley
- ½ cup non-dairy milk
- 1-2 tablespoon almond butter
- 1 teaspoon honey

Blend all ingredients together to the desired consistency. Serve immediately.

30. Sensational Summer in a Glass

A blend of flavorful fruits puts you in the right mood to take on any task, any day.

- 1 banana, sliced and frozen
- 1 kiwi, sliced
- ½ cup strawberries, halved
- ½ cup blueberries
- 3-4 cherries, pitted
- 2 cups assorted leafy greens
- 1 cup fresh-squeezed orange juice
- ice cubes
- mint leaves

Blend the banana, berries, kiwi, cherries, ice and orange juice. Add the greens. Blend to the desired consistency. Garnish with mint and serve immediately.

Weight-Loss Smoothies

31. Banana-Strawberry Dream

When you're craving for something sweet, thick and creamy, try this milkshake-inspired smoothie.

- 1 banana, sliced and frozen
- 1 cup strawberries, halved
- ½ cup fresh coconut meat
- 1 cup spinach
- mint leaves
- ice cubes (optional)

Blend the banana, coconut meat, ice and strawberries together. Add the spinach and blend to the desired consistency. Garnish with mint leaves. Serve immediately.

32. Banana-Mango Cooler

Instead of strawberries, add mangoes to the previous recipe for a tropical twist.

- 1 banana, sliced and frozen
- 1 mango, cubed
- ½ cup fresh coconut meat
- 1 cup spinach
- mint leaves
- ice cubes (optional)

Blend the banana, coconut meat, ice and mangoes together. Add the spinach and blend to the desired consistency. Garnish with mint leaves. Serve immediately.

33. Decadent Detox Smoothie

Flush out toxins and fats with this fruity green smoothie.

- ½ cup pineapple, cubed
- ½ cup blueberries, fresh or frozen
- 2 cups kale
- water

Blend the pineapple and the blueberries with water. Add the kale. Blend to the desired consistency. Serve immediately.

34. Berry Merry Flusher

Deliciously tart and slimming as well.

- 1 cup mixed berries, fresh or frozen
- 1 cup Romaine lettuce
- 1 celery stalk
- water
- 1 tablespoon golden flax seeds

Blend the berries, celery and water together. Add the lettuce and the flax seeds. Blend to the desired consistency. Serve immediately.

35. Gooey Green Goodie

Healthy fats from avocados keep you feeling full, but don't add unwanted pounds.

- 1 avocado, cubed
- 1 ripe pear, cubed

- 2 cups spinach
- 2 tablespoons fresh-squeezed lime juice
- water

Blend the avocado, pear, and water together. Add the spinach and lime juice. Blend to the desired consistency. Serve immediately.

36. Sweet and Sour Spectacular

Berries and oranges perfectly complement each other in this fat-flushing smoothie.

- 1 cup strawberries, halved
- half of a large orange
- 1 cup spinach
- a handful of parsley
- water

Blend the strawberries, orange and water together. Add the spinach and parsley. Blend to the desired consistency. Garnish with a strawberry and serve immediately.

37. Stone Fruit Bonanza
Delight your taste buds with this sweet and tart smoothie.

- 1 nectarine, cubed
- 2 plums, cubed
- 1 peach, cubed
- 1 cup spinach
- a splash of fresh-squeezed orange juice

Blend the nectarine, plums, peach and orange juice together. Add the spinach and pulse some more. Serve immediately.

38. Antioxidation Sensation
Take advantage of the amazing antioxidant property of blueberries.

- 1 cup blueberries, fresh or frozen
- 1 banana, sliced and frozen
- 1 cup kale
- 1 cup almond butter
- 1 teaspoon golden flax seeds

Blend the blueberries and banana together. Add the kale, almond butter and flax seeds. Blend to the desired consistency. Serve immediately.

39. Blissful Melon Smoothie

Did you know that melons contain fewer calories than you burn while you eat it?

- 1 cup melon, cubed
- 1 cup spinach
- 1 tablespoon fresh-squeezed orange juice
- 1 teaspoon chia seeds
- ice cubes

Blend the melon, ice and orange juice together. Add the spinach and the chia seeds. Blend to the desired consistency. Serve immediately.

40. Cucumber-Melon Cooler

This is the perfect all-natural no-sugar-added drink for a hot summer day.

- 1 cup melon, cubed
- 1 small cucumber, cubed
- 1 cup kale or spinach
- 2 basil leaves
- ice cubes

Blend the melon, cucumber, and ice together. Add the greens and pulse some more. Serve immediately.

Metabolism-Boosting Smoothies

41. "Your Favorite Sandwich" Smoothie

Craving for a PB&J? Or a PB&B? Substitute with this.

- 2 bananas, sliced and frozen
- 1 cup spinach
- 6 tablespoons almond butter
- 1 cup almond milk
- 1 tablespoon honey or ½ teaspoon organic coco sugar
- ice cubes

Blend the bananas, almond butter, milk and ice. Add the spinach and sweetener. Blend to the desired consistency. Serve immediately.

42. Asian Pear Smoothie
Pair the crisp sweetness of pear with the unexpected zing of ginger for this unique energizing smoothie.

- 1 pear, cubed
- 1 banana, sliced and frozen
- 1 inch fresh ginger, peeled and grated
- 1 cup assorted leafy greens
- water

Blend the pear, banana, ginger and water together. Add the greens and pulse some more. Serve immediately.

43. Banana-Coconut Delight
This is creamy goodness in a glass.

- 1 banana, sliced and frozen
- 1 cup fresh coconut meat
- 1 cup spinach
- ½ cup coconut milk
- 1 teaspoon golden flax seeds
- 1 teaspoon honey
- ice cubes

Blend the banana, coconut, milk and ice cubes together. Add the spinach, flax seeds and honey. Blend to the desired consistency. Serve immediately.

44. Luscious Berry-Banana Smoothie
Is this creamy, fruity smoothie breakfast or dessert? Perhaps... both!

- 1 banana, sliced and frozen
- 1 cup assorted berries, fresh or frozen
- 1 cup Romaine lettuce
- 1 cup spinach
- 1 celery stalk
- 1 cup almond milk
- 1 teaspoon honey
- 1 teaspoon chia seeds

- ½ teaspoon maca powder
- ice cubes

Blend the banana, berries, celery, milk, and ice together. Add the lettuce, spinach, honey and maca powder. Blend to the desired consistency. Mix in the chia seeds. Serve.

45. Autumn Chill Green Smoothie

The flavors of autumn abound in this comforting glass of seasonal goodness.

- 2 apples, cubed
- 1 cup kale
- 1 cup Romaine lettuce
- 2 Medjool dates, pitted
- 1 cup almond milk
- ½ teaspoon cinnamon
- ¼ teaspoon nutmeg
- 1 teaspoon honey
- ice cubes

Blend the apples, dates, ice and milk together. Add the kale, lettuce, cinnamon, nutmeg and honey. Blend to the desired consistency. Dust with cinnamon and serve immediately.

46. All Hallow's Smoothie

Love pumpkin pie? Then you'll enjoy this tasty pumpkin-based smoothie.

- 1 apple, cubed
- 1 cup homemade pumpkin puree
- 1 cup kale
- 1 cup spinach
- 1 cup almond milk
- 1 teaspoon honey or maple syrup
- ½ teaspoon cinnamon

Blend the apple, pumpkin and milk together. Add the kale, spinach, cinnamon and sweetener. Blend to the desired consistency. Dust with cinnamon and serve.

47. Peach and Almond Not-milkshake

Peaches and almonds are both excellent metabolism-boosters that are rich in essential fatty acids and fiber.

- 2 cups peaches, cubed
- 1 cup Romaine lettuce
- 1 cup almond milk
- 1 tablespoon almond butter
- 1 teaspoon honey (optional)
- ice cubes

Blend the peaches with the almond milk and ice. Add the lettuce, honey and almond butter. Blend to the desired consistency. Serve immediately.

48. Cucumber Basil Lemonade

Cucumber, basil and lemon give your metabolism a jump-start while effectively cleaning your digestive tract.

- 1 cucumber, sliced
- a handful of basil
- 1 cup spinach
- juice of 1 lemon
- 1 tablespoon honey or ½ tablespoon organic coco sugar
- mint leaves
- water
- ice cubes

Blend the cucumber with the water and ice. Add the spinach, basil, lemon juice, sweetener and a mint leaf. Blend to the desired consistency. Garnish with a mint leaf and serve immediately.

49. Supercharging Blackberry Smoothie

Blackberries and pineapples are high in fiber and rich in antioxidants. Spinach improves muscle function, amping up the effect of your workouts.

- 1 cup blackberries, fresh or frozen
- 1/2 cup pineapple, cubed
- 2 cups spinach
- water
- ice cubes

Blend the blackberries, pineapple, water and ice together. Add the spinach and pulse some more. Serve immediately.

50. Heavenly Green Smoothie

Here's another metabolism-boosting smoothie to satisfy your sweet tooth and give you an all-natural mood boost.

- 1 banana, sliced and frozen
- 1 apple, cubed
- 1/2 cup pineapple, cubed
- 1 cup Romaine lettuce
- 1 cup spinach
- a handful of parsley
- ½ cup fresh-squeezed orange juice
- ½ cup almond milk
- ice cubes

Blend the banana, apple, pineapple, almond milk, orange juice and ice together. Add the spinach, lettuce and parsley. Blend to the desired consistency. Serve immediately.

Chapter 9: Smoothie-Making Basics

It should go without saying, but just to be clear: do *not* buy green smoothies from chain juice bars, food courts and fast food chains. Mixing up homemade green smoothies is the only way to ensure that you are getting the real deal, made with care in a clean setting from fresh, all-natural ingredients.

Here are a few more easy tips and tricks to making green smoothies.

How to prepare your green smoothie:

- Purchase your fruits and greens at the farmer's market. Make sure that you get produce that is fresh, whole, in season, organic, and locally grown. Stay away from pre-packaged and/or processed fruits and vegetables. Except in the cases of certain flash-frozen produce, these have already lost most of their nutrient content and may contain artificial color and toxic preservatives.
- When you get home, give your fruits and vegetables a vinegar bath. Just add a tablespoon or two of organic apple cider vinegar to a basin of water and soak fruits and vegetables for at least 10 minutes to get rid of dirt, as well as pesticides and fertilizers that may have contaminated your market haul.
- Getting the proper equipment is important. Though you don't really need to buy an expensive blender like the Vitamix, do make sure that you get a high-speed blender with an 800-watt motor.
- If you are not using a high-speed blender, then process the tougher ingredients (fruits, chunkier vegetables, ice) with liquids (water, juice, non-dairy milk alternative) before adding the softer ones (leafy greens).
- If you're always in a rush in the morning, cut up fruits and vegetables the night before and store individual portions in freezer bags. In the morning, grab a bag and dump the contents into the blender. Whizz and pour into portable tumblers.
- Remember that when it comes to green smoothies, the simpler the better. Ideally, green smoothies should only

contain vegetables, fruits and water. However, you may add other ingredients depending on the purpose of your green smoothie.

- Do not add starchy vegetables to your green smoothie.

How to drink your green smoothie:

- Take your green smoothie in the morning, on an empty stomach. This is the best way for the body to fully absorb all the nutrients in your smoothie. Taking it this way also amps up the smoothie's cleansing and detoxifying properties.
- Sip green smoothies slowly instead of gulping them down. Swirl it around your mouth, letting it mix with your saliva, before swallowing.

How to store your green smoothie:

- To reap the maximum amount of nutrients from your green smoothie, make sure to consume it immediately. However, you can store leftovers in the freezer. Thaw and drink these within three days.
- Turn leftover green smoothies into green pops by pouring the smoothie into Popsicle molds and freezing it. This is a great way of feeding little ones their daily allowance of fruits and vegetables.

Chapter 10: Tips For Making Your Smoothie Taste Great

- For those on a vegan or a vegetarian diet, almond milk, hemp milk, soy milk, rice milk, and coconut milk are excellent non-dairy milk alternatives.
- Use frozen bananas to give your green smoothie the texture of a milkshake. Peel ripe bananas, slice them up and stash them in the freezer. Frozen bananas are also great for making the simplest dessert ever – one-ingredient vegan ice cream!
- Add nut butters, coconut milk, or coconut meat for extra creamy smoothies.
- If you are not fond of thick smoothies, then add more liquid or reduce the amount of bananas in the recipe. When making banana-based green smoothies, try to consume the smoothie as soon as possible because the bananas will make it *really* thick while it sits in your glass.
- Health food supplements make your green smoothie even more nutritious than it already is. Maca powder, moringa powder, spirulina, golden flax seeds, hemp seeds, sunflower kernels, chia seeds, goji berries, virgin coconut oil, and many other superfoods are incorporated well into green smoothies and even impart their own unique flavors to the drinks.
- Try many different recipes and you will eventually discover what works for you and what doesn't. Tweak recipes to suit your taste buds. When you see an unfamiliar fruit or vegetable in the market, bring it home and see if you can use it in your smoothies. Dare to experiment! Have fun in the kitchen!

Conclusion

Thank you again for purchasing this book on the Green Smoothie Diet!

I am extremely excited to pass this information along to you, and I am so happy that you now have read and can hopefully implement these strategies going forward.

I hope this book was able to help you understand green smoothies and the benefits of a daily green smoothie habit. I hope you have also learned how to integrate green smoothies into your everyday life, how to properly make and store them, and how to make sure that you keep this habit for your optimum health and wellbeing.

The next step is to get started using this information and to hopefully live a healthier, more nourished, less disease-prone, stress-free, energetic, and rejuvenated life!

Please don't be someone who just reads this information and doesn't apply it. The strategies in this book will only benefit you if you use them!

If you know of anyone else that could benefit from the information presented here please inform them of this book.

Finally, if you enjoyed this book and feel it has added value to your life in any way, please take the time to share your thoughts and post a review on Amazon. It'd be greatly appreciated!

Thank you and good luck!

Preview Of:

Ultimate Carb Cycling Guide!

<u>Carb Cycling</u>

Quickly Lose Fat, Preserve Muscle Mass, And Build Self Confidence With Sustainable Fat Loss Carb Cycling Diet Tips And Strategies That Work Fast!

Introduction

I want to thank you and congratulate you for purchasing the book, *Carb Cycling: Ultimate Carb Cycling Guide! - Quickly Lose Fat, Preserve Muscle Mass, And Build Self Confidence With Sustainable Fat Loss Carb Cycling Diet Tips And Strategies That Work Fast!*

This book contains proven steps and strategies on how to plan your own carb cycling diet with explanations of the concept, the science behind it, and several food recommendations.

Have you heard of cyclic ketogenic diet? No? Well, that isn't a bad thing. You probably already know about it, more popularly known as carb cycling.

To keep one's body fit, there are a lot of things to consider. One of those is attaining an ideal weight. If you already have an ideal weight, then it's just a matter of maintaining it. If you're overweight, then you have to reduce weight. If you're underweight, then you should gain weight. But you shouldn't just stop with the numbers you see on the weighing scale. Your body's composition is also important. When losing or gaining weight, you must be sure that you are losing fat and gaining muscle.

Two things play the greatest part here: diet and physical activity. Weight is about the calories: how much you get from the food you eat and how much you spend on the physical things you do. There should be a correct balance between them. Diet and exercise go hand in hand in this matter. Although these two things can be discussed together, our main focus here is dieting.

Thanks again for purchasing this book, I hope you enjoy it!

Chapter 1: Understand The Concept Of Carb Cycling

There have been a lot of diets formulated since long ago. You probably heard of many whether you've been searching or not. To a certain extent, all of them can work since diet is basically calorie deficit. Consume less than what you spend and you lose weight. The thing is that a healthy weight is not just about the quantity but also the quality. It is not just how much you eat that matters, but also the kind of food you eat. Diet can get a little complicated especially if you have further goals such as building and toning your muscles or gaining an ideal body for a specific sport.

Carb cycling is one of the many diets popular among body-builders and athletes. That's because it can build and maintain muscle mass. Also, it adds efficiency in fat burning.

Carb cycling may have its roots from bodybuilding but now it gained significance even in the general health community. That explains a good part of why it's getting a great deal of attention nowadays. Since you're reading this book, it's quite likely that it got your attention, too. You probably want an in-depth learning of carb cycling. So, let's finish up this introduction and get to the good part: learning about carb cycling and how to apply it.

In order to effectively apply carb cycling into your own lifestyle, you must understand deeply its concept. As mentioned earlier, the science behind the diet can get really complicated. But don't worry. You don't really need to go into all the technical terms and whatnot in order to understand carb cycling, or any diet for that matter. This book will still discuss the science behind carb cycling but it can be simplified enough for the average person.

What is carb cycling?

Controlling carbohydrate intake has been of great importance when talking about nutrition. Studies abound regarding the relation of improper carbohydrate intake to serious health concerns such as chronic diseases and obesity. But still, carbohydrates are also important for our body. So, it is not always just about reducing the carbohydrates you consume, but actually taking in the right amount of carbohydrates.

The above is the reason why carb cycling and similar diets were formed. The carb cycling diet uses an approach of alternating the level of carbohydrate consumption. Such a diet involves periods of zero, low and high carbohydrate intake. As it turns out, it isn't just about taking in the right kind and amount of carbohydrates but also taking them at the right time. The kind of carbohydrates, how much, and when you will take them influence how your body responds to them.

In a carb cycling diet, you schedule your week into no-carb, low-carb, and high-carb days. Note that a high-carb day doesn't mean you'll pig out on carbs – you still control the amount but just higher compared to the other days. You'll see more on that later.

A carb cycling diet doesn't only take carbs into consideration. There's also protein and fat – taking the right amount of these is equally important. Throughout the schedule, you need a high level of protein intake. For fat, it is inversely proportional to your carb intake. Thus, during zero or low-carb days, your fat intake should be high. During high-carb days, you consume low fat.

Carb cycling diets will be varied in terms of specific protocols. However, they all share the same basis. The structure is simple: a few days of low-carbs, one day of high-carbs, followed by a day of zero-carbs or low-carbs, and the cycle goes back to the beginning.

As an example, you may schedule four consecutive days of low-carb, high-carb the next day, zero-carb after that, and back to the beginning. Or, schedule three consecutive days of low-carb, one high-carb day, and then back to low-carb.

To gain insight on what is involved in a carb cycling diet, here are some numerical figures:

- On a high-carb day, your set amount of carbohydrate intake is generally between 2 to 2.5 grams for every pound of body weight. Protein intake is set at 1 gram for every pound while fat intake is set to 0 to 0.15 grams for every pound.

- On a moderate-carb day, carbohydrate intake is 1.5 grams for every pound. Protein is at 1 to 1.2 grams for every pound, and fat is at 0.2 grams for every pound.

- On a low-carb day, the intake is at 1.5 grams of carbohydrates for each pound of weight. Protein intake is generally increased to around 1.5 grams per body pound, and fat goes up to 0.35 grams for every pound.

- A zero-carb or no-carb day doesn't really mean zero carbohydrates at all. The term is just for distinguishing from the low-carb since the no-carb day has a really low limit. It no longer takes into consideration body weight – you must not go over 30 grams of carbohydrates for the whole day. Here, you consume 1.5 grams of protein for every pound and fat rises up to 0.5 to 0.8 grams for every pound. Note that this zero/no-carb day is skipped by some people. It is up to your goals or what fits your level of physical activity.

As you can see, the diet involves a detailed measurement of the carbohydrates, protein, and fat that you consume. It takes a lot of discipline especially if you have specific goals. You must really get into the diet if you want to accomplish it. However, once you start, you'll find that it is not as difficult to incorporate to your daily lifestyle compared to other types of diet. Furthermore, this book is a good starting point.

Thanks for Previewing My Exciting Book Entitled:

"Carb Cycling: Ultimate Carb Cycling Guide! Quickly Lose Fat, Preserve Muscle Mass, And Build Self Confidence With Sustainable Fat Loss Carb Cycling Diet Tips And Strategies That Work Fast!"

To purchase this book, simply go to the Amazon Kindle store and simply search:

"CARB CYCLING"

Then just scroll down until you see my book. You will know it is mine because you will see my name "Chris Smith" underneath the title.

Alternatively, you can visit my author page on Amazon to see this book and other work I have done. Thanks so much, and please don't forget your free bonuses

DON'T LEAVE YET! - CHECK OUT YOUR FREE BONUSES BELOW!

Free Bonus Offer: Get Free Access To The www.LiveFitVIP.com VIP Newsletter!

Once you enter your email address you will immediately get free access to this awesome newsletter!

But wait, right now if you join now for free you will also get free access to the "The 7 Keys To Body Transformation" free EBook!

To claim both your FREE VIP NEWSLETTER MEMBERSHIP and your FREE BONUS EBook on THE 7 KEYS TO BODY TRANSFORMATION!

Just Go To:

www.liveFitVIP.com

www.ingramcontent.com/pod-product-compliance
Lightning Source LLC
Chambersburg PA
CBHW070840290526
45795CB00002B/932